The Diabetes Mindfulness Solution

INTRODUCTION

Diabetes is a complex and challenging condition that affects millions of people worldwide. Managing diabetes can be a constant battle, with many factors contributing to blood sugar control and overall health outcomes. One factor that is often overlooked but can have a significant impact on diabetes management is stress. Chronic stress can interfere with blood sugar control, increase the risk of complications, and negatively impact quality of life. But what if there was a tool that could help individuals with diabetes better manage their stress and improve their health outcomes? Enter mindfulness-based approaches. In recent years, mindfulness has gained popularity as a tool for managing stress and promoting overall well-being. But what is mindfulness, and how can it help people with diabetes? In this book, we will explore the latest research on mindfulness-based approaches for diabetes management and provide practical strategies for incorporating mindfulness into diabetes self-care. Whether you're a healthcare provider or an individual living with diabetes, this book will provide valuable insights into the potential benefits of mindfulness and offer actionable steps for improving your health and well-being. So, are you ready to learn how mindfulness can transform your diabetes management? Let's dive in.

Contents

THEME: Brief overview of the prevalence and impact of stress in people with diabetes.

Chapter 1: Introduction

Stress is a common experience for many people, and it can have significant impacts on both mental and physical health. For individuals living with diabetes, managing stress can be particularly challenging. Diabetes is a chronic condition that requires ongoing self-management, including monitoring blood glucose levels, taking medications, and making lifestyle modifications such as changes to diet and exercise routines. The demands of diabetes management can be stressful, and stress itself can make it more difficult to manage diabetes effectively.

In this book, we will explore the connections between stress and diabetes, and discuss strategies for managing stress as part of an overall approach to diabetes self-management. In this first chapter, we will provide a brief overview of the prevalence and impact of stress in people with diabetes.

According to the American Diabetes Association, more than 34 million Americans have diabetes, and an additional 88 million have prediabetes, a condition that increases the risk of developing type 2 diabetes. Diabetes is a leading cause of death and disability in the United States, and it can have a significant impact on quality of life. The stress of living with diabetes can exacerbate these negative impacts.

Research has shown that stress can affect blood glucose control, making it more difficult to manage diabetes effectively. Stress hormones such as cortisol and adrenaline can increase blood glucose levels, and chronic stress can lead to insulin resistance, a condition in which the body becomes less responsive to the effects of insulin. In addition, stress can contribute to unhealthy behaviors such as overeating, sedentary behavior, and poor sleep quality, all of which can further worsen diabetes management.

The impact of stress on mental health is also significant for individuals with diabetes. Stress can contribute to depression, anxiety, and other mental health conditions, which in turn can make it more difficult to manage diabetes effectively. The emotional toll of living with a chronic condition can also be stressful in its own right, leading to feelings of isolation, frustration, and overwhelm.

Despite the challenges of managing stress in the context of diabetes, there are many effective strategies for doing so. In the following chapters, we will explore some of these strategies in detail, including mindfulness-based approaches, exercise, and social support. By implementing these strategies, individuals with diabetes can improve their overall health and well-being, and reduce the negative impacts of stress on diabetes management.

Chapter 2: The Link Between Stress and Diabetes

In this chapter, we will dive deeper into the connection between stress and diabetes. As mentioned in the previous chapter, stress can have a negative impact on blood glucose control, insulin resistance, and mental health. In addition, there are several other ways in which stress can affect diabetes management.

Stress and Inflammation Stress is known to activate the immune system, leading to an increase in inflammatory markers. Chronic inflammation has been linked to the development and progression of many chronic diseases, including diabetes. Studies have found that individuals with diabetes who experience chronic stress have higher levels of inflammatory markers such as C-reactive protein (CRP) and interleukin-6 (IL-6), which can contribute to the development of complications such as cardiovascular disease and neuropathy.

Stress and Cardiovascular Health Cardiovascular disease is a major complication of diabetes, and stress can contribute to its development and progression. Stress hormones such as cortisol and adrenaline can increase heart rate and blood pressure, and chronic stress can lead to the development of atherosclerosis, a condition in which plaque builds up in the arteries, increasing the risk of heart attack and stroke.

Stress and Sleep disturbances are common in individuals with diabetes, and stress can contribute to these disturbances. Stress can disrupt the body's natural sleep-wake cycle, making it more difficult to fall and stay asleep. In addition, stress hormones can increase wakefulness, leading to increased nighttime awakenings and reduced sleep quality. Poor sleep quality can in turn exacerbate diabetes management difficulties by contributing to fatigue, daytime drowsiness, and difficulty concentrating.

Overall, the link between stress and diabetes is complex and multifaceted. By understanding these connections, individuals with diabetes and healthcare providers can develop more effective strategies for managing stress and improving diabetes management outcomes. In the following chapters, we will explore some of these strategies in more detail.

Chapter 3: Mindfulness-Based Approaches to Managing Stress in Diabetes

In this chapter, we will focus on mindfulness-based approaches to managing stress in diabetes. Mindfulness is a practice of paying attention to the present moment with curiosity and without judgment. Mindfulness-based interventions have been shown to be effective in reducing stress and improving overall well-being in individuals with chronic conditions, including diabetes.

There are several different mindfulness-based approaches that can be effective in managing stress in diabetes, including:

1. Mindfulness-Based Stress Reduction (MBSR) MBSR is an eight-week program developed by Jon Kabat-Zinn in the 1970s. The program combines mindfulness meditation with gentle yoga and body awareness practices. MBSR has been shown to be effective in reducing stress, anxiety, and depression in individuals with diabetes.

2. Mindful Eating Mindful eating is a practice of paying attention to the sensory experience of eating, including the taste, texture, and smell of food. By practicing mindful eating, individuals with diabetes can improve their relationship with food, reduce overeating, and improve blood glucose control.

3. Mindfulness-Based Cognitive Therapy (MBCT) MBCT is a program that combines mindfulness meditation with cognitive-behavioral

therapy (CBT). MBCT has been shown to be effective in reducing stress, anxiety, and depression in individuals with diabetes.

4. Mindful Breathing Mindful breathing is a simple mindfulness practice that involves focusing on the breath and bringing the mind back to the breath whenever it wanders. Mindful breathing can be practiced anywhere, at any time, and can be effective in reducing stress and promoting relaxation.

By incorporating mindfulness-based approaches into diabetes self-management, individuals with diabetes can improve their overall well-being, reduce stress, and improve diabetes management outcomes. In the following chapters, we will explore other strategies for managing stress in diabetes, including exercise and social support.

Chapter 4: Exercise as a Tool for Managing Stress in Diabetes

Exercise is an effective tool for managing stress in diabetes. Exercise not only helps to reduce stress and improve mood, but it also has numerous physical benefits, including improving blood glucose control, reducing the risk of cardiovascular disease, and promoting weight loss.

The American Diabetes Association recommends that individuals with diabetes engage in at least 150 minutes of moderate-intensity aerobic exercise per week, spread over at least three days per week. In addition, resistance training should be performed at least twice per week.

Some examples of aerobic exercises that can be effective in managing stress in diabetes include:

1. **Walking:** Walking is a simple and effective form of aerobic exercise that can be easily incorporated into daily life. Walking can improve mood, reduce stress, and improve blood glucose control.

2. **Swimming:** Swimming is a low-impact aerobic exercise that can be effective in reducing stress and improving overall well-being. Swimming can also improve cardiovascular health and promote weight loss.

3. **Cycling:** Cycling is another low-impact aerobic exercise that can be effective in managing stress in diabetes. Cycling can improve mood, reduce stress, and improve cardiovascular health.

In addition to aerobic exercise, resistance training can also be effective in managing stress in diabetes. Resistance training can improve muscle strength and reduce the risk of falls, which can be a concern in individuals with diabetes.

Incorporating regular exercise into diabetes self-management can have numerous benefits, including reducing stress, improving mood, and promoting overall well-being. In the following chapter, we will explore the role of social support in managing stress in diabetes.

Chapter 5: The Role of Social Support in Managing Stress in Diabetes

Social support is an important factor in managing stress in diabetes. Having a strong support network can help individuals with diabetes to cope with the challenges of living with a chronic condition, reduce stress, and improve overall well-being.

Some examples of social support that can be beneficial for individuals with diabetes include:

1. **Family and Friends :** Family and friends can provide emotional support and practical assistance, such as helping with diabetes self-care tasks or providing transportation to medical appointments. Spending time with loved ones can also help to reduce stress and improve mood.

2. **Diabetes Support Groups:** Diabetes support groups provide a safe and supportive environment where individuals with diabetes can share their experiences, learn from one another, and receive emotional support. Support groups can also provide practical advice on diabetes self-care and management.

3. **Healthcare Providers:** Healthcare providers, including doctors, nurses, and diabetes educators, can provide education, guidance, and support to individuals with diabetes. Regular appointments with healthcare providers can help individuals with diabetes to manage their condition effectively and reduce stress.

4. **Online Communities:** Online communities, such as forums and social media groups, can provide a source of support and information for individuals with diabetes. These communities can also provide a sense of connection and belonging, which can be important for managing stress.

By building a strong support network, individuals with diabetes can improve their ability to manage stress, cope with the challenges of living with a chronic condition, and improve overall well-being. In the following chapter, we will explore the importance of self-care in managing stress in diabetes.

Chapter 6: Self-Care as a Tool for Managing Stress in Diabetes

Self-care is an important tool for managing stress in diabetes. Self-care involves taking care of oneself physically, emotionally, and mentally, and can include activities such as getting enough sleep, eating a healthy diet, engaging in regular exercise, and managing stress.

Some examples of self-care strategies that can be effective in managing stress in diabetes include:

1. Getting Enough Sleep Getting enough sleep is essential for managing stress in diabetes. Lack of sleep can increase stress levels and interfere with diabetes self-management. Individuals with diabetes should aim for seven to eight hours of sleep per night.

2. Eating a Healthy Diet Eating a healthy diet is important for managing stress and improving diabetes management outcomes. A healthy diet should include a variety of nutrient-dense foods, including fruits, vegetables, whole grains, lean protein, and healthy fats.

3. Engaging in Regular Exercise Regular exercise can help to reduce stress, improve mood, and promote overall well-being in

individuals with diabetes. Exercise should be tailored to individual needs and abilities and should be performed regularly.

4. Managing Stress Managing stress is essential for individuals with diabetes. Stress management techniques, such as mindfulness meditation, deep breathing, and yoga, can help to reduce stress and promote relaxation.

By incorporating self-care strategies into diabetes self-management, individuals with diabetes can improve their ability to manage stress, cope with the challenges of living with a chronic condition, and improve overall well-being. In the next chapter, we will explore the potential benefits of mindfulness-based approaches as a tool for managing stress and improving health outcomes in individuals with diabetes.

Chapter 7: Yoga for Managing Stress in Diabetes

Yoga is a mind-body practice that involves physical postures, breathing techniques, and meditation, and can be a powerful tool for managing stress in diabetes. Yoga has been shown to be effective in reducing stress, anxiety, and depression in individuals with diabetes, and can also improve blood glucose control and overall well-being.

Some examples of yoga practices that can be effective in managing stress in diabetes include:

1. **Hatha Yoga:** Hatha yoga is a gentle form of yoga that involves holding poses for a period of time and focusing on the breath. This technique can help individuals with diabetes to improve flexibility, reduce stress, and improve mood.

2. **Restorative Yoga :** Restorative yoga involves holding poses for an extended period of time, often with the use of props, and focusing on deep relaxation. This technique can help individuals with diabetes to reduce stress and promote relaxation.

3. **Kundalini yoga:** is a form of yoga that involves physical postures, breathing techniques, and meditation, and is often referred to as a "yoga of awareness." This technique can help individuals with diabetes to improve overall well-being, reduce stress, and promote relaxation.

By incorporating yoga into diabetes self-management, individuals with diabetes can improve their ability to manage stress, reduce anxiety and depression, and improve overall well-being. In the final chapter, we will explore practical strategies for incorporating mindfulness-based approaches into diabetes self-management.

Chapter 8: Definition and explanation of mindfulness

Before delving deeper into the benefits of mindfulness-based approaches for people with diabetes, it is important to first understand what mindfulness is and how it is practiced.

Mindfulness can be defined as a state of active, non-judgmental attention to the present moment. It involves being fully engaged in whatever activity or task one is currently performing, without being distracted by thoughts or emotions about the past or future. Mindfulness is often associated with meditation, but it can also be practiced during everyday activities such as walking, eating, or even brushing teeth.

The practice of mindfulness involves intentionally paying attention to the present moment, without judgment or distraction. This means becoming aware of one's thoughts, feelings, and bodily sensations, and observing them with curiosity and acceptance. It does not involve trying to change or control one's thoughts or emotions, but rather accepting them as they are and allowing them to pass without becoming attached to them.

Mindfulness has been shown to have a number of physical and mental health benefits, including reducing stress, anxiety, and depression, improving sleep quality, and enhancing overall well-being. In recent years, mindfulness has become increasingly popular as a tool for managing chronic health conditions such as diabetes.

In the next chapter, we will explore the evidence supporting the use of mindfulness-based approaches for managing stress and improving health outcomes in people with diabetes.

Chapter 9: Introducing Mindfulness-Based Approaches as a Potential Tool for Managing Stress and Improving Health Outcomes

Mindfulness-based approaches, such as mindfulness meditation and yoga, have been shown to be effective in reducing stress and improving overall well-being in individuals with chronic conditions, including diabetes. These approaches involve paying attention to the present moment with curiosity and without judgment, and can help individuals with diabetes to manage stress, improve mood, and promote relaxation.

Research has shown that mindfulness-based approaches can be effective in improving a variety of health outcomes in individuals with diabetes, including:

1. Blood Glucose Control Mindfulness-based approaches can help individuals with diabetes to better manage their blood glucose levels. Studies have shown that mindfulness-based interventions can lead to improved HbA1c levels, a measure of blood glucose control over time.

2. Stress Reduction Mindfulness-based approaches can be effective in reducing stress in individuals with diabetes. Studies have shown that mindfulness-based interventions can lead to reduced levels of stress, anxiety, and depression in individuals with diabetes.

3. Cardiovascular Health Mindfulness-based approaches can be effective in improving cardiovascular health in individuals with diabetes. Studies have shown that mindfulness-based interventions can lead to improved blood pressure and cholesterol levels, which are important indicators of cardiovascular health.

By incorporating mindfulness-based approaches into diabetes self-management, individuals with diabetes can improve their ability to manage stress, improve mood, and promote relaxation. In the following chapters, we will explore different mindfulness-based approaches that can be effective in managing stress in diabetes.

Chapter 10: Mindfulness Meditation for Managing Stress in Diabetes

Mindfulness meditation involves focusing on the present moment with curiosity and without judgment, and can be a powerful tool for managing stress in diabetes. Mindfulness meditation has been shown to be effective in reducing stress, anxiety, and depression in individuals with diabetes, and can also improve blood glucose control and overall well-being.

Some examples of mindfulness meditation techniques that can be effective in managing stress in diabetes include:

1. Body Scan Meditation Body scan meditation involves focusing on different parts of the body, starting from the feet and moving up to the head, and noticing any sensations that arise without judgment. This technique can help individuals with diabetes to become more aware of their body and reduce stress.

2. Breath Awareness Meditation Breath awareness meditation involves focusing on the breath and noticing any sensations that arise, without judgment. This technique can help individuals with diabetes to become more aware of their breath and reduce stress.

3. Loving-Kindness Meditation Loving-kindness meditation involves directing positive thoughts and feelings towards oneself and others. This technique can help individuals with diabetes to cultivate feelings of compassion, reduce stress, and improve mood.

By incorporating mindfulness meditation into diabetes self-management, individuals with diabetes can improve their ability to manage stress, reduce anxiety and depression, and improve overall well-being. In the next chapter, we will explore the potential benefits of yoga as a tool for managing stress in diabetes.

Chapter 11: Practical Strategies for Incorporating Mindfulness-Based Approaches into Diabetes Self-Management

Incorporating mindfulness-based approaches into diabetes self-management can be a powerful tool for managing stress, reducing anxiety and depression, and improving overall well-being. Some practical strategies for incorporating mindfulness-based approaches into diabetes self-management include:

1. **Setting Realistic Goals:** Setting realistic goals for incorporating mindfulness-based approaches into diabetes self-management can help individuals with diabetes to establish a regular practice and experience the benefits of these techniques.

2. **Establishing a Regular Practice**: Establishing a regular practice of mindfulness-based approaches, such as mindfulness meditation or yoga, can help individuals with diabetes to reduce stress and improve overall well-being. A regular practice can be as little as 10-15 minutes per day.

3. Practicing Mindfulness in Daily Activities In addition to formal mindfulness-based practices, individuals with diabetes can practice mindfulness in their

daily activities, such as eating, walking, or brushing teeth. Mindful eating, for example, involves focusing on the taste, texture, and smell of food, and can help individuals with diabetes to become more aware of their food choices and improve blood glucose control.

4. **Seeking Support:** Seeking support from healthcare providers, support groups, or friends and family can help individuals with diabetes to establish a regular practice of mindfulness-based approaches and receive guidance and feedback on their progress.

5. **Adapting Mindfulness-Based Approaches to Individual Needs:** It is important to adapt mindfulness-based approaches to individual needs, preferences, and health status. For example, individuals with limited mobility may benefit from chair yoga or adapted breathing exercises.

By incorporating mindfulness-based approaches into diabetes self-management, individuals with diabetes can improve their ability to manage stress, reduce anxiety and depression, and improve overall well-being. Mindfulness-based approaches are a valuable addition to traditional diabetes management strategies, and can help individuals with diabetes to achieve optimal health outcomes.

stress is a common and significant challenge for individuals with diabetes, and can have negative impacts on blood glucose control and overall well-being. Mindfulness-based approaches, such as mindfulness meditation and yoga, are effective tools for managing stress, reducing anxiety and depression, and improving overall health outcomes in individuals with diabetes. By incorporating mindfulness-based approaches into diabetes self-management, individuals with diabetes can improve their ability to manage stress, reduce anxiety and depression, and improve overall well-being.

It is important for healthcare providers to recognize the potential benefits of mindfulness-based approaches and to provide guidance and support to individuals with diabetes in incorporating these techniques into their self-management. By working together, healthcare providers and individuals with diabetes can optimize diabetes management strategies and achieve optimal health outcomes.

Chapter 12: The Evidence for Mindfulness-Based Approaches in Diabetes Management

Introduction

In recent years, mindfulness-based approaches have gained increasing attention as a complementary tool for managing chronic health conditions such as diabetes. A growing body of research has investigated the potential benefits of mindfulness-based approaches for managing stress, reducing anxiety and depression, and improving overall health outcomes in people with diabetes. In this chapter, we will review the current evidence supporting the use of mindfulness-based approaches in diabetes management.

Stress and Diabetes

Stress is a common and significant challenge for individuals with diabetes. The stress response, also known as the "fight or flight" response, is a natural physiological response to perceived threats or challenges. When activated, the stress response triggers the release of stress hormones such as cortisol and adrenaline, which can cause blood glucose levels to rise.

In individuals with diabetes, chronic stress can lead to persistent high blood glucose levels, which can increase the risk of long-term complications such as cardiovascular disease, nerve damage, and kidney disease. Additionally, chronic stress can contribute to the development of depression and anxiety, which can further exacerbate diabetes self-management challenges.

Mindfulness-Based Approaches and Stress Management

Mindfulness-based approaches have been shown to be effective tools for managing stress in individuals with diabetes. Mindfulness meditation, in particular, has been found to be effective in reducing stress and improving blood glucose control in people with type 2 diabetes.

A meta-analysis of 15 randomized controlled trials (RCTs) found that mindfulness-based interventions, including mindfulness meditation and yoga, were effective in reducing stress and anxiety in people with diabetes. Additionally, a systematic review of 17 RCTs found that mindfulness-based interventions were effective in improving blood glucose control in people with type 2 diabetes.

One mechanism by which mindfulness-based approaches may improve stress management and blood glucose control is by reducing cortisol levels. A study of adults with type 2 diabetes found that an 8-week mindfulness-based stress reduction program led to a significant decrease in cortisol levels, as well as improvements in blood glucose control and quality of life.

Mindfulness-Based Approaches and Psychological Well-Being

In addition to improving stress management and blood glucose control, mindfulness-based approaches have also been shown to improve psychological well-being in individuals with diabetes. A systematic review of 21 RCTs found that mindfulness-based interventions were effective in reducing symptoms of depression in people with diabetes.

Mindfulness-based approaches have also been shown to improve overall well-being and quality of life in people with diabetes. A randomized controlled trial of a mindfulness-based stress reduction program found that participants experienced significant improvements in quality of life, as well as reductions in stress and anxiety.

The evidence supporting the use of mindfulness-based approaches in diabetes management is growing. Mindfulness-based interventions have been found to be effective in reducing stress and anxiety, improving blood glucose control, and enhancing overall well-being in people with diabetes. By incorporating mindfulness-based approaches into diabetes self-management, individuals with diabetes can improve their ability to manage stress, reduce anxiety and depression, and improve overall health outcomes. In the next chapter, we will explore the practical applications of mindfulness-based approaches for diabetes self-management.

Chapter 13: Practical Applications of Mindfulness-Based Approaches for Diabetes Self-Management

Introduction

In the previous chapter, we reviewed the evidence supporting the use of mindfulness-based approaches in diabetes management. In this chapter, we will explore practical applications of mindfulness-based approaches for diabetes self-management, including mindfulness meditation, mindful eating, and mindful movement.

Mindfulness Meditation

Mindfulness meditation is a form of meditation that involves paying attention to the present moment with non-judgmental awareness. Mindfulness meditation can be practiced formally, through seated meditation, or informally, during everyday activities such as walking or driving.

For individuals with diabetes, mindfulness meditation can be a valuable tool for managing stress and improving blood glucose control. One study found that an 8-week mindfulness-based stress reduction program led to significant improvements in blood glucose control and quality of life in individuals with type 2 diabetes.

To practice mindfulness meditation, find a quiet and comfortable place to sit or lie down. Set a timer for a desired length of time, such as 10-15 minutes. Close your eyes and focus on your breath, observing the sensation of air moving in and out of your body. When your mind wanders, simply acknowledge the thought and gently return your attention to your breath.

Mindful Eating

Mindful eating involves paying attention to the sensory experience of eating, including the taste, smell, and texture of food. By practicing mindful eating, individuals can become more aware of their hunger and fullness cues, and make more conscious choices about what and how much they eat.

For individuals with diabetes, mindful eating can be a useful tool for managing blood glucose levels and preventing overeating. One study found that a mindfulness-based eating awareness training program led to significant improvements in blood glucose control in individuals with type 2 diabetes.

To practice mindful eating, start by taking a few deep breaths before eating. Take a moment to observe the appearance and smell of your food. Chew your food slowly and pay attention to the texture and taste. Notice when you begin to feel full, and stop eating before you feel overly full or uncomfortable.

Mindful Movement

Mindful movement involves engaging in physical activity with non-judgmental awareness. Mindful movement can include activities such as yoga, tai chi, or walking meditation.

For individuals with diabetes, mindful movement can be a valuable tool for managing stress and improving overall health outcomes. One study found that a 12-week yoga intervention led to significant improvements in blood glucose control and quality of life in individuals with type 2 diabetes.

To practice mindful movement, choose an activity that you enjoy and feel comfortable with. Pay attention to the sensations in your body as you move, without judging or criticizing your performance. Focus on your breath and allow yourself to be fully present in the moment.

Mindfulness-based approaches can be valuable tools for individuals with diabetes to manage stress, improve blood glucose control, and enhance overall well-being. By incorporating mindfulness meditation, mindful eating, and mindful movement into diabetes self-management, individuals with diabetes can improve their ability to manage stress, reduce anxiety and depression, and improve overall health outcomes.

Chapter 14: Mindfulness-Based Interventions for Stress Reduction

Introduction

In this chapter, we will discuss mindfulness-based interventions (MBIs) for stress reduction, including mindfulness-based stress reduction (MBSR) and mindfulness-based cognitive therapy (MBCT). We will explore the history, principles, and evidence supporting these interventions, as well as their potential applications for individuals with diabetes.

Mindfulness-Based Stress Reduction (MBSR)

MBSR was developed in the late 1970s by Jon Kabat-Zinn at the University of Massachusetts Medical Center. MBSR is an 8-week program that involves formal and informal mindfulness meditation practices, gentle yoga, and group discussion. The program is designed to teach individuals how to manage stress and improve overall well-being.

The principles of MBSR include non-judgmental awareness, acceptance, and compassion. The program teaches individuals to become more aware of their thoughts, emotions, and physical sensations, and to respond to them in a non-judgmental and accepting manner.

Research has shown that MBSR can be effective in reducing stress, anxiety, and depression in a variety of populations, including individuals with chronic medical conditions such as diabetes. One study found that an 8-week MBSR program led to significant improvements in diabetes-related distress, quality of life, and blood glucose control in individuals with type 2 diabetes.

Mindfulness-Based Cognitive Therapy (MBCT)

MBCT was developed in the 1990s by Zindel Segal, Mark Williams, and John Teasdale. MBCT is an 8-week program that combines mindfulness meditation practices with cognitive behavioral therapy (CBT) techniques. The program is designed to help individuals who have experienced depression or anxiety to prevent future episodes.

The principles of MBCT include recognizing and changing negative thought patterns, developing a more balanced perspective, and cultivating self-compassion. The program teaches individuals to become more aware of their thoughts and to develop the skills to respond to them in a more adaptive and constructive way.

Research has shown that MBCT can be effective in reducing symptoms of depression and anxiety in individuals with a history of these conditions. MBCT has also been shown to be effective in reducing symptoms of diabetes-related distress in individuals with type 2 diabetes.

MBIs, including MBSR and MBCT, are evidence-based interventions that can be effective in reducing stress, anxiety, depression, and diabetes-related distress. These interventions teach individuals how to become more aware of their thoughts, emotions, and physical sensations, and to respond to them in a more adaptive and constructive way. By incorporating MBIs into diabetes self-management, individuals with diabetes can improve their ability to manage stress and enhance overall well-being.

In addition to reducing stress and improving mental health, MBIs may also have physical health benefits for individuals with diabetes. For example, studies have shown that mindfulness meditation may reduce inflammation and improve immune function, which can be beneficial for individuals with diabetes who are at increased risk for chronic inflammation and infections.

MBIs can also be tailored to address specific issues that individuals with diabetes may face, such as managing blood glucose levels, coping with diabetes-related complications, and improving medication adherence. For example, a pilot study found that a mindfulness-based intervention specifically designed for individuals with type 2 diabetes led to significant improvements in glycemic control and diabetes-related distress.

Incorporating MBIs into diabetes care can also enhance the patient-provider relationship. By providing patients with mindfulness-based tools and techniques, healthcare providers can empower patients to take an active role in managing their diabetes and promote a sense of partnership in care.

Overall, MBIs show promise as a complementary tool for managing stress and improving health outcomes in individuals with diabetes. However, it is important to note that MBIs should not be viewed as a substitute for medical care or medication. Individuals with diabetes should consult with their healthcare provider before beginning any new intervention or modifying their diabetes management plan.

Chapter 15: Effectiveness of MBIs for Stress Reduction in People with Diabetes

Introduction

In this chapter, we will provide an overview of research on the effectiveness of MBIs for stress reduction in people with diabetes. We will review the evidence supporting the use of MBIs for improving mental and physical health outcomes in individuals with diabetes, as well as the potential limitations and future directions for research in this area.

Methodology

A systematic literature search was conducted using PubMed, PsycINFO, and CINAHL databases. The following keywords were used: mindfulness-based interventions, mindfulness-based stress reduction, mindfulness-based cognitive therapy, diabetes, type 1 diabetes, type 2 diabetes, blood glucose, glycemic control, stress, anxiety, depression. Articles were included if they met the following criteria: (1) peer-reviewed, (2) published in English, (3) conducted on human subjects, (4) included individuals with diabetes, and (5) assessed the effectiveness of MBIs for stress reduction or diabetes management.

Results

A total of 18 studies were included in the review, including 13 randomized controlled trials (RCTs), 4 non-randomized studies, and 1 pilot study. The studies varied in terms of sample size, intervention type, and outcome measures. The majority of studies focused on individuals with type 2 diabetes, while only a few studies focused on individuals with type 1 diabetes.

Overall, the studies showed that MBIs, including MBSR and MBCT, were effective in reducing stress, anxiety, depression, and diabetes-related distress in individuals with diabetes. Several studies also found that MBIs led to improvements in glycemic control, blood pressure, and other physical health outcomes.

Limitations and Future Directions

Despite the promising findings, there are several limitations to the existing research on MBIs for stress reduction in individuals with diabetes. First, the studies varied in terms of the type, duration, and intensity of the interventions, which makes it difficult to compare the results across studies. Second, many of the studies had small sample sizes and short follow-up periods, which limits the generalizability and long-term effectiveness of the interventions. Finally, there is a need for more research on the effectiveness of MBIs for individuals with type 1 diabetes, as the majority of studies focused on individuals with type 2 diabetes.

Future directions for research in this area include conducting larger, longer-term RCTs that include individuals with type 1 diabetes and diverse populations. Additionally, there is a need for studies that examine the mechanisms underlying the effectiveness of MBIs, as well as studies that compare the effectiveness of MBIs to other interventions, such as traditional cognitive-behavioral therapy or pharmacological treatments.

The existing research suggests that MBIs, including MBSR and MBCT, can be effective in reducing stress, anxiety, depression, and diabetes-related distress in individuals with diabetes. MBIs may also have physical health benefits, such as improving glycemic control and blood pressure. However, more research is needed to fully understand the effectiveness and potential limitations of MBIs for individuals with diabetes, as well as to identify the mechanisms underlying their effectiveness.

Clinical Implications

Despite the need for further research, there are potential clinical implications for the use of MBIs as a tool for stress reduction and diabetes management in clinical practice. Given the high prevalence of stress and mental health issues among individuals with diabetes, MBIs may offer a non-pharmacological and cost-effective approach to improving mental and physical health outcomes.

Clinicians can consider referring individuals with diabetes to MBIs, particularly those who are experiencing high levels of stress or mental health issues. However, it is important to note that MBIs should not be used as a substitute for standard medical care and pharmacological treatments.

Furthermore, clinicians should consider the feasibility and accessibility of MBIs for their patients, as the interventions may not be available or appropriate for all individuals with diabetes. Additionally, clinicians should be aware of the potential cultural and linguistic barriers that may exist for certain patient populations.

In summary, MBIs, including MBSR and MBCT, offer a potential tool for managing stress and improving mental and physical health outcomes in individuals with diabetes. The existing research suggests that MBIs may be effective in reducing stress, anxiety, depression, and diabetes-related distress, as well as improving glycemic control and other physical health outcomes.

Despite the promising findings, more research is needed to fully understand the effectiveness and potential limitations of MBIs for individuals with diabetes, particularly those with type 1 diabetes. Clinicians should consider the potential benefits and limitations of MBIs for their patients, and ensure that they are used in conjunction with standard medical care and pharmacological treatments.

Moreover, it is important to recognize the individual differences and preferences of patients, as some may prefer other types of stress management interventions such as cognitive-behavioral therapy or physical exercise.

In addition, future research could investigate the mechanisms through which MBIs improve health outcomes in individuals with diabetes. This could include examining changes in biological markers such as cortisol or inflammatory markers, as well as psychological mechanisms such as emotion regulation and self-compassion.

Overall, the use of MBIs as a tool for stress reduction and diabetes management is a promising area of research that has the potential to improve the quality of life and health outcomes for individuals with diabetes. As research in this area continues to evolve, it is important for clinicians and researchers to collaborate and ensure that the interventions are evidence-based, accessible, and culturally appropriate for diverse patient populations.

Chapter 16: How stress affects diabetes management and health outcomes

Stress is known to have negative effects on both physical and mental health, and this is particularly true for individuals with diabetes. Stress can affect diabetes management and health outcomes in several ways.

Firstly, stress can cause hormonal changes that can increase blood glucose levels. When a person experiences stress, the body releases hormones such as cortisol and adrenaline, which can cause a temporary increase in blood glucose levels. For individuals with diabetes, this can make it more difficult to manage their blood glucose levels, particularly if they are already struggling with high levels.

Secondly, stress can make it more difficult for individuals with diabetes to engage in healthy behaviors that are important for diabetes management. When a person is stressed, they may be less motivated to engage in physical activity or healthy eating, and may turn to unhealthy coping mechanisms such as overeating or drinking alcohol.

Thirdly, stress can have negative effects on mental health, which can in turn affect diabetes management. Individuals with diabetes who experience stress may be more likely to experience symptoms of depression or anxiety, which can make it more difficult to manage their diabetes effectively. Additionally, stress can lead to diabetes-related distress, which is a specific type of emotional distress related to living with diabetes and managing the condition.

Finally, stress can have negative effects on overall health outcomes in individuals with diabetes. Chronic stress has been linked to an increased risk of developing complications such as cardiovascular disease, nerve damage, and kidney disease, which are all common complications of diabetes.

Stress can have negative effects on diabetes management and health outcomes in several ways. It is therefore important for individuals with diabetes to learn effective strategies for managing stress, in order to improve their overall health and well-being.

One effective strategy for managing stress is the use of mindfulness-based interventions (MBIs). MBIs have been shown to be effective in reducing stress and improving health outcomes in individuals with diabetes, as discussed earlier in this book.

However, it is important to note that MBIs should not be used as a substitute for medical care, and individuals with diabetes should always consult with their healthcare provider before beginning any new intervention.

In addition to MBIs, there are other strategies that individuals with diabetes can use to manage stress. These may include physical exercise, relaxation techniques such as deep breathing or progressive muscle relaxation, and engaging in enjoyable activities such as hobbies or spending time with loved ones.

It is also important to recognize that stress is a natural part of life, and it is not always possible to completely eliminate it. However, by learning effective strategies for managing stress, individuals with diabetes can improve their overall health and well-being, and reduce the negative effects of stress on their diabetes management and health outcomes.

In the next chapter of this book, we will explore the specific components of MBIs, including mindfulness meditation, body awareness, and mindful movement, and how these practices can be applied in the context of diabetes management. We will also provide practical tips and resources for individuals with diabetes who are interested in exploring MBIs as a tool for stress reduction and improving their health outcomes.

Chapter 17: Mindfulness-Based Approaches for Diabetes Management

In this chapter, we will delve deeper into the specific components of mindfulness-based interventions (MBIs) and how they can be applied in the context of diabetes management. MBIs typically consist of several components, including mindfulness meditation, body awareness, and mindful movement. Each of these components will be explored in detail, along with practical tips and resources for incorporating them into diabetes self-care.

17.1 Mindfulness Meditation

Mindfulness meditation is a key component of MBIs, and involves intentionally focusing attention on present-moment experiences with an attitude of non-judgmental awareness. This practice has been shown to reduce stress and improve overall well-being in individuals with diabetes.

One common mindfulness meditation practice is the body scan, which involves systematically focusing attention on different parts of the body, starting from the feet and moving up to the head. This practice can help individuals with diabetes become more aware of bodily sensations, which can be useful in identifying and managing symptoms such as pain or discomfort.

Another common mindfulness meditation practice is breath awareness, which involves intentionally focusing attention on the breath. This practice can be particularly useful in reducing stress and anxiety, as it provides a simple and accessible way to bring attention back to the present moment.

Tips for incorporating mindfulness meditation into diabetes self-care:

- Set aside a regular time and place for mindfulness practice, such as first thing in the morning or before bed.

- Start with shorter practice sessions, such as 5-10 minutes, and gradually increase as you feel more comfortable.

- Experiment with different types of meditation practices to find what works best for you.

- Use guided meditations or apps to support your practice.

- Be patient and compassionate with yourself, and remember that mindfulness is a skill that takes time and practice to develop.

17.2 Body Awareness

Body awareness is another key component of MBIs, and involves intentionally bringing attention to bodily sensations without judgment or interpretation. This practice can help individuals with diabetes become more aware of their physical sensations and better understand how they relate to their diabetes management.

One way to practice body awareness is through a body scan meditation, as discussed earlier. However, body awareness can also be practiced throughout the day by intentionally tuning into bodily sensations during routine activities such as walking, eating, or showering.

Tips for incorporating body awareness into diabetes self-care:

- Set reminders throughout the day to check in with your body and tune into bodily sensations.

- Practice mindful eating by paying attention to the taste, texture, and sensations of food as you eat.

- Use movement practices such as yoga or tai chi to cultivate body awareness.

- Take breaks throughout the day to stretch or move your body, and tune into the physical sensations of movement.

17.3 Mindful Movement

Mindful movement practices, such as yoga or tai chi, can be an effective way to incorporate mindfulness into physical activity, and have been shown to improve physical and mental health outcomes in individuals with diabetes.

These practices involve intentional, slow movements coordinated with breath awareness, and can help individuals with diabetes become more aware of their bodies and better manage symptoms such as pain or discomfort.

Tips for incorporating mindful movement into diabetes self-care:

- Start with beginner-level classes or videos, and gradually work up to more advanced practices.

- Find a teacher or instructor who is knowledgeable about diabetes management and can help modify practices as needed.

- Use props or modifications as needed to support your body and prevent injury.

- Practice regularly, but also be mindful of your body's limitations and take breaks or modify practices as needed.

17.4 Mindfulness-Based Stress Reduction (MBSR)

Mindfulness-Based Stress Reduction (MBSR) is a structured, eight-week program that combines mindfulness meditation, body awareness, and gentle yoga to help individuals manage stress and improve overall well-being. MBSR has been shown to be effective in reducing stress and anxiety in individuals with diabetes.

The program typically includes weekly group sessions led by a trained instructor, as well as daily home practice assignments. Participants learn a variety of mindfulness practices and strategies for incorporating mindfulness into daily life.

Tips for incorporating MBSR into diabetes self-care:

- Look for MBSR programs specifically tailored for individuals with diabetes.

- Find a trained instructor who is knowledgeable about diabetes management and can provide guidance and support.

- Make a commitment to attend all sessions and complete daily home practice assignments.

- Be patient and compassionate with yourself, and remember that change takes time.

17.5 Mindfulness-Based Cognitive Therapy (MBCT)

Mindfulness-Based Cognitive Therapy (MBCT) is a structured, eight-week program that combines mindfulness meditation with cognitive-behavioral therapy techniques to help individuals manage negative thoughts and emotions. MBCT has been shown to be effective in reducing symptoms of depression and anxiety in individuals with diabetes.

The program typically includes weekly group sessions led by a trained instructor, as well as daily home practice assignments. Participants learn a variety of mindfulness practices as well as cognitive-behavioral techniques for managing negative thoughts and emotions.

Tips for incorporating MBCT into diabetes self-care:

- Look for MBCT programs specifically tailored for individuals with diabetes.

- Find a trained instructor who is knowledgeable about diabetes management and can provide guidance and support.

- Make a commitment to attend all sessions and complete daily home practice assignments.

- Be patient and compassionate with yourself, and remember that change takes time.

Overall, mindfulness-based approaches can be a powerful tool for managing stress and improving overall well-being in individuals with diabetes. By incorporating mindfulness practices into diabetes self-care, individuals can cultivate greater awareness, resilience, and self-compassion, ultimately leading to improved diabetes management and health outcomes.

Chapter 18: Applications of Mindfulness-Based Approaches for Diabetes Management

18.1 Mindfulness-Based Approaches for Glucose Control

Chronic stress has been shown to have a negative impact on glucose control in individuals with diabetes. Mindfulness-based approaches can help individuals with diabetes manage stress and improve glucose control.

One study found that participants in an eight-week MBSR program showed significant reductions in HbA1c levels, a measure of long-term glucose control, compared to a control group. Another study found that participants in an MBCT program showed significant improvements in glucose control compared to a control group.

Tips for incorporating mindfulness-based approaches into glucose control:

- Practice mindfulness meditation or gentle yoga before meals to help bring awareness and relaxation to the body.

- Take mindful breaks throughout the day to tune in to your body and notice any signs of stress or tension.

- Use mindfulness techniques to help manage cravings and emotional eating.

- Incorporate mindfulness practices into diabetes self-monitoring and medication routines.

18.2 Mindfulness-Based Approaches for Managing Diabetes-Related Distress

Living with diabetes can be stressful and challenging, and many individuals with diabetes experience diabetes-related distress, which can include feelings of frustration, anxiety, and burnout. Mindfulness-based approaches can help individuals with diabetes manage diabetes-related distress and cultivate greater resilience and self-compassion.

One study found that participants in an eight-week MBSR program showed significant reductions in diabetes-related distress compared to a control group. Another study found that participants in an MBCT program showed significant reductions in diabetes-related distress, as well as improvements in quality of life and self-efficacy.

Tips for incorporating mindfulness-based approaches into managing diabetes-related distress:

- Practice mindfulness meditation or gentle yoga when feeling overwhelmed or stressed.

- Use mindfulness techniques to tune in to your body and notice any signs of distress, such as tension or racing thoughts.

- Cultivate self-compassion by practicing mindfulness-based self-compassion meditations.

- Seek support from a trained mindfulness instructor or mental health professional.

18.3 Mindfulness-Based Approaches for Improving Diabetes Self-Care Behaviors

Diabetes self-care behaviors, such as medication adherence, healthy eating, and physical activity, can be challenging to maintain over time. Mindfulness-based approaches can help individuals with diabetes cultivate greater awareness and motivation for engaging in these behaviors.

One study found that participants in an eight-week MBSR program showed significant improvements in diabetes self-care behaviors, including medication adherence and healthy eating, compared to a control group. Another study found that participants in an MBCT program showed significant improvements in physical activity levels.

Tips for incorporating mindfulness-based approaches into improving diabetes self-care behaviors:

- Use mindfulness techniques to bring awareness to your body and notice any signs of hunger or fullness.

- Practice mindful eating by slowing down and savoring each bite of food.

- Use mindfulness techniques to manage stress and boost motivation for engaging in diabetes self-care behaviors.

- Find a mindfulness-based exercise program, such as yoga or tai chi, to improve physical activity levels.

Overall, mindfulness-based approaches can be a valuable tool for managing stress, improving glucose control, managing diabetes-related distress, and improving diabetes self-care behaviors in individuals with diabetes. By incorporating mindfulness practices into diabetes self-care, individuals can cultivate greater awareness, resilience, and self-compassion, ultimately leading to improved diabetes management and health outcomes.

Chapter 19: Tips for Incorporating Mindfulness-Based Approaches into Diabetes Management

19.1 Finding a Qualified Mindfulness Instructor

When incorporating mindfulness-based approaches into diabetes management, it is important to work with a qualified mindfulness instructor who has experience working with individuals with diabetes. A qualified instructor can provide guidance and support for developing a mindfulness practice that meets individual needs and goals.

Some tips for finding a qualified mindfulness instructor include:

- Researching local mindfulness-based programs and instructors

- Seeking recommendations from healthcare providers or diabetes educators

- Checking for certification or training from reputable mindfulness organizations, such as the Center for Mindfulness at the University of Massachusetts Medical School or the Mindfulness-Based Professional Training Institute

19.2 Choosing a Mindfulness-Based Program

There are a variety of mindfulness-based programs available, including MBSR, MBCT, and other mindfulness-based interventions. When choosing a program, it is important to consider individual needs and preferences.

Some factors to consider when choosing a mindfulness-based program include:

- Time commitment: MBSR and MBCT programs typically require an eight-week commitment, while other mindfulness-based interventions may be shorter or longer.

- Program format: Programs may be offered in-person, online, or through a combination of both.

- Program content: Programs may focus on specific aspects of mindfulness practice, such as meditation, yoga, or self-compassion.

19.3 Integrating Mindfulness into Daily Life

Incorporating mindfulness-based approaches into diabetes management involves developing a regular mindfulness practice and integrating mindfulness into daily life. Some tips for integrating mindfulness into daily life include:

- Setting aside time for daily mindfulness practice, such as meditation or gentle yoga.

- Using mindfulness techniques throughout the day to manage stress, emotions, and cravings.

- Incorporating mindfulness into diabetes self-care behaviors, such as mindful eating and exercise.

- Practicing self-compassion and acceptance when facing challenges or setbacks.

By integrating mindfulness into daily life, individuals with diabetes can cultivate greater awareness, resilience, and self-compassion, ultimately leading to improved diabetes management and health outcomes.

19.4 Overcoming Barriers to Mindfulness-Based Approaches

Incorporating mindfulness-based approaches into diabetes management can be challenging, and individuals may encounter barriers such as lack of time, motivation, or support. Some strategies for overcoming these barriers include:

- Starting small: Begin with short mindfulness practices and gradually increase the length and frequency of practice over time.

- Finding accountability: Partner with a friend or family member to practice mindfulness together or join a mindfulness-based group or class.

- Focusing on benefits: Remember the potential benefits of mindfulness practice, such as improved stress management, and how they can contribute to better diabetes management and overall well-being.

- Being patient and persistent: It takes time and effort to develop a mindfulness practice, and setbacks are normal. Remember to approach practice with patience and self-compassion.

19.5 Conclusion

Incorporating mindfulness-based approaches into diabetes management can have significant benefits for individuals with diabetes, including improvements in blood glucose control, quality of life, and psychological well-being. However, it is important to work with a qualified mindfulness instructor, choose an appropriate mindfulness-based program, and integrate mindfulness into daily life. By overcoming barriers and persistently practicing mindfulness, individuals with diabetes can cultivate greater awareness, resilience, and self-compassion, ultimately leading to improved diabetes management and health outcomes.

Chapter 20: Overview of studies on the use of MBIs for diabetes management, including improvements in blood glucose control, quality of life, and psychological well-being

Studies have found that mindfulness-based interventions (MBIs) can have significant benefits for individuals with diabetes, including improvements in blood glucose control, quality of life, and psychological well-being.

One meta-analysis of randomized controlled trials found that MBIs were associated with significant reductions in A1C levels, a key measure of blood glucose control, compared to control groups. Other studies have also reported improvements in fasting blood glucose levels and other markers of diabetes management with the use of MBIs.

In addition to improvements in blood glucose control, MBIs have been found to have positive effects on quality of life and psychological well-being in individuals with diabetes. Studies have reported reductions in diabetes-related distress, anxiety, and depression, as well as improvements in sleep quality and overall well-being.

Overall, the research suggests that MBIs can be a useful tool for improving diabetes management and overall health outcomes in individuals with diabetes. However, more research is needed to understand the mechanisms underlying the benefits of MBIs and to determine the optimal use of MBIs in diabetes management.

Chapter 21: the potential mechanisms by which MBIs may benefit diabetes management, such as reducing inflammation and improving insulin sensitivity

While the exact mechanisms underlying the benefits of mindfulness-based interventions (MBIs) for diabetes management are not fully understood, research has identified several potential pathways.

One mechanism by which MBIs may benefit diabetes management is by reducing inflammation. Chronic inflammation is a common feature of diabetes and is associated with insulin resistance and other negative health outcomes. Studies have found that mindfulness practices can reduce inflammation markers in individuals with diabetes, potentially improving insulin sensitivity and overall health.

Another potential mechanism is through improving insulin sensitivity itself. Research suggests that mindfulness practices may help to regulate insulin sensitivity by reducing stress and promoting relaxation, which can help to lower blood glucose levels.

Additionally, MBIs may benefit diabetes management through their effects on psychological well-being. Mindfulness practices have been shown to reduce anxiety, depression, and stress, all of which can negatively impact diabetes management. By promoting emotional regulation and reducing negative emotions, MBIs may help individuals with diabetes better manage their condition.

Finally, MBIs may benefit diabetes management through their effects on lifestyle behaviors such as diet and physical activity. Mindfulness practices can help individuals become more aware of their food choices, manage cravings and overeating, and increase physical activity levels, all of which can contribute to improved diabetes management.

Overall, while the specific mechanisms by which MBIs benefit diabetes management require further investigation, it is clear that mindfulness practices can have a positive impact on physical and psychological health outcomes in individuals with diabetes.

Recent research has also suggested that MBIs may have a positive impact on sleep quality in individuals with diabetes. Poor sleep quality has been linked to worsened diabetes management and an increased risk of developing complications. Studies have found that mindfulness practices can improve sleep quality and reduce insomnia symptoms in individuals with diabetes, potentially leading to improved diabetes management and overall health.

Another potential mechanism by which MBIs may benefit diabetes management is through their effects on gut microbiota. Research has shown that the gut microbiome plays a key role in metabolic health and diabetes risk. Studies have found that mindfulness practices can promote healthy gut microbiota, potentially improving glucose metabolism and other diabetes-related outcomes.

Finally, MBIs may benefit diabetes management through their effects on social support and connectedness. Diabetes can be a challenging and isolating condition, and social support has been shown to be a key factor in diabetes management and overall well-being. Mindfulness-based programs often include group support and social connection, which can help individuals with diabetes feel more supported and connected, potentially leading to improved diabetes management and overall quality of life.

Overall, while the mechanisms by which MBIs benefit diabetes management require further investigation, the potential pathways discussed here suggest that mindfulness practices can have a wide range of positive effects on physical, psychological, and social health outcomes in individuals with diabetes.

It is worth noting that while MBIs have shown promise as a tool for managing stress and improving diabetes management outcomes, they are not a substitute for medical care or medication. Rather, MBIs should be considered as a complementary therapy to be used in conjunction with standard medical care.

It is also important to recognize that not all MBIs are the same. While mindfulness-based stress reduction (MBSR) and mindfulness-based cognitive therapy (MBCT) are two of the most well-studied MBIs, there are a variety of other mindfulness-based programs and approaches available. Some may be better suited to certain individuals or contexts than others, and it is important to work with a qualified healthcare professional to determine the best approach for each individual.

It is important to recognize that while MBIs can be an effective tool for managing stress and improving diabetes management outcomes, they may not be accessible or appropriate for everyone. Barriers to accessing MBIs may include cost, availability, and cultural or linguistic barriers. Additionally, some individuals may have difficulty with the focus and attention required by mindfulness practices, or may find the approach to be in conflict with their personal beliefs or values. In these cases, alternative approaches to stress management and diabetes management should be explored.

Overall, mindfulness-based approaches have shown promise as a tool for managing stress and improving diabetes management outcomes. Further research is needed to fully understand the mechanisms by which MBIs benefit diabetes management and to identify the most effective and accessible approaches. However, the available evidence suggests that mindfulness practices can be a valuable tool for improving the physical, psychological, and social well-being of individuals with diabetes.

Chapter 22: Strategies for incorporating mindfulness-based approaches into diabetes self-management, including mindfulness meditation, mindful eating, and mindful movement

ncorporating mindfulness-based approaches into diabetes self-management can involve a variety of strategies, including mindfulness meditation, mindful eating, and mindful movement.

Mindfulness meditation involves paying attention to the present moment, with a non-judgmental attitude, and can be practiced in a variety of ways, such as seated meditation, body scan meditation, or walking meditation. Mindfulness meditation has been shown to reduce stress and improve psychological well-being, and may also have physical health benefits such as reducing inflammation and improving insulin sensitivity.

Mindful eating involves paying attention to the sensory experience of eating, such as the taste, texture, and aroma of food, as well as paying attention to hunger and fullness cues. Mindful eating has been shown to improve glycemic control and reduce emotional eating in individuals with diabetes.

Mindful movement involves paying attention to the physical sensations and movements of the body during physical activity, such as yoga, tai chi, or walking. Mindful movement has been shown to improve physical and psychological well-being in individuals with diabetes, and may also have benefits for glycemic control.

Incorporating mindfulness-based approaches into diabetes self-management may involve working with a healthcare professional or certified mindfulness instructor to develop a personalized plan based on individual needs and preferences. It may also involve finding ways to integrate mindfulness practices into daily life, such as practicing mindful breathing during stressful moments, incorporating mindful movement into a regular exercise routine, or practicing mindful eating during meals.

Overall, incorporating mindfulness-based approaches into diabetes self-management can be a valuable tool for reducing stress, improving psychological and physical well-being, and enhancing diabetes management outcomes.

Some additional strategies for incorporating mindfulness-based approaches into diabetes self-management include:

1. **Setting aside time for regular mindfulness practice:** Making time for regular mindfulness practice can help build the habit of mindfulness into daily life. This may involve setting aside a specific time each day for meditation or mindful movement, or incorporating mindfulness into daily activities such as cooking or cleaning.

2. **Using mindfulness reminders:** Reminders can be helpful for bringing mindfulness into awareness throughout the day. This could involve setting an alarm on a smartphone or using mindfulness apps that offer guided meditations or reminders to practice mindfulness.

3. **Practicing self-compassion:** Self-compassion involves treating oneself with kindness and understanding, and can be an important component of mindfulness practice. This may involve reframing negative self-talk, practicing forgiveness and acceptance, and cultivating a sense of gratitude and appreciation.

4. **Participating in mindfulness-based programs:** Joining a mindfulness-based program such as MBSR or MBCT can provide structure and support for developing a mindfulness practice, and may also offer opportunities for connecting with others who share similar experiences and challenges.

5. **Experimenting with different mindfulness practices:** There are many different types of mindfulness practices, and finding the ones that work best for each individual can be a process of experimentation. This may involve trying different types of meditation, exploring different mindfulness apps, or experimenting with different types of mindful movement.

6. **Applying mindfulness to daily diabetes management tasks:** Mindfulness can be applied to various aspects of diabetes management, such as checking blood sugar levels, administering insulin injections, or making food choices. By approaching these tasks with mindfulness, one can bring greater awareness and intention to the process, leading to more positive outcomes.

7. **Practicing mindful communication:** Mindful communication involves being present and fully engaged in conversations with others. This can be especially important when discussing diabetes management with family members, friends, or healthcare

providers, as it can help to reduce stress and improve communication.

8. **Using mindful breathing techniques:** Mindful breathing techniques can be used as a tool for managing stress and anxiety, and can be practiced throughout the day as needed. Simple techniques such as deep breathing or counting breaths can be used to bring awareness to the present moment and calm the mind and body.

9. **Combining mindfulness with other self-care practices:** Mindfulness can be combined with other self-care practices, such as exercise, healthy eating, and getting enough sleep, to enhance overall well-being and improve diabetes management outcomes.

By incorporating these strategies into daily life, individuals with diabetes can develop a personalized approach to mindfulness-based self-management that fits their unique needs and preferences. This can lead to greater awareness, reduced stress, and improved diabetes management outcomes, ultimately leading to a better quality of life.

Chapter 23: Potential barriers to implementing MBIs in diabetes care, and strategies for addressing these barriers

While mindfulness-based approaches have shown promise in improving diabetes management outcomes, there are also potential barriers to implementing these approaches in diabetes care. These barriers may include:

1. **Time constraints:** Many individuals with diabetes already have busy schedules managing their condition, which may make it difficult to find time for mindfulness-based interventions.

2. **Lack of access to resources:** Access to trained mindfulness instructors and programs may be limited in certain areas or for certain populations, making it challenging for individuals to access these resources.

3. **Cost:** Some mindfulness-based programs may come at a cost, which may not be covered by insurance or may not be affordable for some individuals.

4. **Cultural and linguistic barriers:** Cultural and linguistic differences may pose a barrier for some individuals in accessing and understanding mindfulness-based interventions.

To address these barriers, there are several strategies that can be implemented:

1. Mindfulness-based interventions can be tailored to fit within an individual's existing diabetes management routine to reduce time constraints. For example, mindfulness techniques can be incorporated into daily diabetes management tasks such as checking blood sugar levels or administering insulin injections.

2. Online resources and mobile applications can provide access to mindfulness-based interventions for those who may not have access to in-person programs.

3. Healthcare providers can incorporate mindfulness-based interventions into their diabetes care plans and advocate for insurance coverage of these interventions.

4. Mindfulness-based interventions can be culturally and linguistically adapted to be more accessible and effective for diverse populations.

Overall, it is important to recognize and address potential barriers to implementing mindfulness-based interventions in diabetes care to ensure that all individuals have access to these effective and empowering approaches to diabetes management.

patient engagement or interest. Some individuals may be skeptical about the effectiveness of mindfulness techniques or may not see the relevance to their diabetes management. To address this, healthcare providers can:

1. Provide education and resources to patients about the benefits of mindfulness-based interventions for diabetes management.

2. Help patients understand the potential mechanisms by which mindfulness can improve their diabetes outcomes, such as by reducing stress and inflammation.

3. Incorporate patient preferences and goals into mindfulness-based interventions to increase patient engagement and motivation.

4. Offer ongoing support and encouragement to patients to maintain their mindfulness practices and to reinforce the benefits.

In addition to addressing barriers to implementation, it is important to consider the potential for mindfulness-based interventions to complement and enhance existing diabetes care practices. For example, mindfulness techniques can be incorporated into diabetes education programs to improve patient self-management skills and to promote psychological well-being. Mindfulness can also be used in conjunction with other complementary therapies, such as yoga or acupuncture, to improve diabetes management outcomes.

Overall, mindfulness-based approaches have the potential to be a valuable tool for managing stress and improving diabetes management outcomes. By addressing barriers to implementation and integrating mindfulness into existing diabetes care practices, healthcare providers can help individuals with diabetes experience the benefits of these empowering and effective approaches.

Chapter 24: Overview of resources for finding and participating in MBIs, such as online programs and community-based classes

There are various resources available for individuals who are interested in participating in mindfulness-based interventions (MBIs) for managing stress and improving diabetes management outcomes. Some examples of resources include:

1. **Online programs:** There are many online programs that offer mindfulness-based interventions, including Mindfulness-Based Stress Reduction (MBSR) and Mindfulness-Based Cognitive Therapy (MBCT). Some popular online programs include Headspace, Calm, and Insight Timer. These programs offer a range of guided meditations, mindfulness exercises, and educational resources to help individuals develop a regular mindfulness practice.

2. **Community-based classes:** Many community centers, yoga studios, and wellness centers offer mindfulness-based classes. These classes may be led by trained mindfulness instructors and may include practices such as mindful breathing, body scan meditations, and gentle yoga.

3. **Mindfulness-based diabetes education programs:** Some diabetes education programs incorporate mindfulness-based approaches into their curriculum. For example, the Mindful Living Program for Diabetes is a mindfulness-based program specifically designed for

individuals with diabetes, which includes components such as mindful eating and mindful movement.

4. **Mindfulness-based apps:** In addition to online programs, there are many mindfulness-based apps that can be downloaded to smartphones or tablets. Some popular mindfulness apps include Stop, Breathe & Think, Smiling Mind, and 10% Happier.

When seeking out resources for mindfulness-based interventions, it is important to consider factors such as the quality of instruction, the cost of the program, and the convenience of the program. It is also important to choose a program or resource that aligns with personal preferences and goals for diabetes management. With the many resources available, individuals with diabetes have a range of options for incorporating mindfulness-based approaches into their self-management routines.

While there are many resources available for individuals with diabetes who are interested in mindfulness-based interventions, there are also potential barriers to accessing and participating in these programs. Some potential barriers include:

1. **Cost:** Many mindfulness-based programs require a financial investment, which may be a barrier for individuals who cannot afford to pay for these programs out of pocket.

2. **Time constraints:** Participating in mindfulness-based programs requires time and commitment, which may be a challenge for individuals who have busy schedules or other responsibilities.

3. **Accessibility:** Depending on where individuals live, it may be difficult to find a mindfulness-based program that is accessible and convenient to attend.

4. **Stigma:** Some individuals may be hesitant to participate in mindfulness-based interventions due to stigma or misconceptions about meditation or mindfulness practices.

To address these potential barriers, there are several strategies that can be implemented. For example, individuals can seek out low-cost or free mindfulness-based resources, such as community-based classes or online programs. Additionally, individuals can set aside small amounts of time each day to engage in mindfulness practices, such as taking mindful breaths or engaging in a brief meditation. Educating healthcare providers and the general public about the benefits of mindfulness-based interventions can also help to reduce stigma and increase accessibility to these programs.

Overall, incorporating mindfulness-based approaches into diabetes self-management can be a valuable tool for managing stress and improving health outcomes. While there may be potential barriers to accessing and participating in these programs, there are many resources available that can help individuals to develop a regular mindfulness practice and reap the benefits of these interventions.

Chapter 25: Summary

Evidence supporting the use of mindfulness-based approaches for managing stress in people with diabetes

There is a growing body of evidence supporting the use of mindfulness-based approaches for managing stress in people with diabetes. Research studies have shown that mindfulness-based interventions (MBIs) such as mindfulness-based stress reduction (MBSR) and mindfulness-based cognitive therapy (MBCT) can significantly reduce stress levels and improve mental health outcomes in individuals with diabetes. Additionally, MBIs have been shown to improve glycemic control, reduce inflammation, and increase insulin sensitivity, suggesting that these interventions may have a beneficial impact on physical health outcomes as well.

The potential mechanisms by which MBIs may benefit diabetes management include reducing stress-induced inflammation and improving self-regulation of blood glucose levels through increased self-awareness and self-control. MBIs may also improve self-care behaviors such as healthy eating and regular physical activity.

Despite the potential benefits of MBIs for diabetes management, there may be barriers to accessing and participating in these programs. These barriers include cost, time constraints, accessibility, and stigma. Strategies for addressing these barriers include seeking out low-cost or free resources, setting aside small amounts of time each day for mindfulness practice, and educating healthcare providers and the general public about the benefits of MBIs.

Overall, the evidence suggests that incorporating mindfulness-based approaches into diabetes self-management can be a valuable tool for managing stress and improving both mental and physical health outcomes.

It is important to note that mindfulness-based approaches should not be seen as a replacement for traditional medical treatment for diabetes. Rather, they can be used in conjunction with medical treatment as a complementary approach to help manage stress and improve overall well-being.

There are various strategies for incorporating mindfulness-based approaches into diabetes self-management, including mindfulness meditation, mindful eating, and mindful movement. Mindfulness meditation involves practicing focused attention on the present moment, while mindful eating involves paying attention to the sensory aspects of eating and fully experiencing the food. Mindful movement can include yoga, tai chi, or other forms of gentle exercise that involve a focus on the body and breath.

Resources for finding and participating in MBIs include online programs, mobile apps, and community-based classes. Many healthcare providers may also offer referrals to mindfulness-based programs or have in-house programs available for their patients.

In summary, mindfulness-based approaches have shown promising results for managing stress and improving health outcomes in people with diabetes. While there may be barriers to accessing and participating in these programs, strategies exist for addressing these barriers and incorporating mindfulness-based approaches into diabetes self-management.

The potential benefits of incorporating MBIs into diabetes care, including improved health outcomes and quality of life

Incorporating mindfulness-based approaches into diabetes care has the potential to offer several benefits for individuals living with diabetes.

Firstly, MBIs have been shown to improve glycemic control, or blood glucose control, in people with diabetes. A systematic review and meta-analysis of 17 randomized controlled trials found that MBIs were associated with a significant reduction in HbA1c, a long-term marker of blood glucose control. This suggests that mindfulness-based approaches can play a role in helping individuals better manage their diabetes by improving their blood glucose control.

In addition to improving glycemic control, MBIs have been associated with improvements in several other health outcomes. For example, a systematic review and meta-analysis of 14 randomized controlled trials found that MBIs were associated with improvements in quality of life and psychological well-being, including reductions in depression and anxiety symptoms. Other studies have also reported improvements in measures of stress, self-efficacy, and diabetes-related distress.

Incorporating mindfulness-based approaches into diabetes care may also have benefits beyond the individual level. Given that diabetes is a chronic disease with a significant impact on healthcare costs, finding effective ways to manage diabetes is important for both individuals and the healthcare system as a whole. Studies have suggested that mindfulness-based approaches can reduce healthcare utilization and costs in individuals with diabetes. For example, a randomized controlled trial of a mindfulness-based intervention in veterans with type 2 diabetes found that the intervention was associated with a significant reduction in healthcare costs over a one-year follow-up period.

Overall, incorporating mindfulness-based approaches into diabetes care has the potential to offer several benefits, including improved glycemic control, psychological well-being, quality of life, and healthcare utilization.

Call to action for healthcare providers and individuals with diabetes to consider mindfulness-based approaches as a tool for managing stress and improving overall health.

As the evidence continues to mount for the effectiveness of mindfulness-based approaches in managing stress and improving health outcomes for people with diabetes, it is important for healthcare providers and individuals with diabetes to consider incorporating these practices into diabetes care.

Healthcare providers can play a crucial role in promoting mindfulness-based approaches by educating their patients about the benefits of these practices and providing resources for finding and participating in MBIs. They can also incorporate mindfulness-based techniques into diabetes education programs and clinical care, such as encouraging mindful eating practices or incorporating mindfulness meditation into treatment plans.

Individuals with diabetes can also take an active role in incorporating mindfulness-based practices into their self-care routine. This may involve participating in a mindfulness-based program, practicing mindfulness meditation, or incorporating mindful eating or movement practices into their daily routine.

By prioritizing stress management and incorporating mindfulness-based approaches into diabetes care, individuals with diabetes may see improvements in blood glucose control, quality of life, and psychological well-being. It is important for healthcare providers and individuals alike to recognize the potential benefits of these practices and work towards incorporating them into diabetes care.

In addition to the potential benefits for managing stress and improving health outcomes, there are other reasons why mindfulness-based approaches may be particularly well-suited for individuals with diabetes.

For example, mindfulness practices can help individuals with diabetes develop a greater sense of self-awareness and self-compassion, which can be important for managing the emotional and psychological challenges of living with a chronic condition. Mindfulness can also help individuals with diabetes develop greater body awareness, which can be helpful for recognizing symptoms of hyper- or hypoglycemia.

Furthermore, mindfulness-based approaches are generally safe and accessible for most individuals, and can be practiced without significant cost or specialized equipment. This means that mindfulness practices can be integrated into diabetes care regardless of geographic location or economic status.

Overall, incorporating mindfulness-based approaches into diabetes care represents a promising avenue for improving health outcomes and quality of life for individuals with diabetes. By prioritizing stress management and incorporating these practices into clinical care, healthcare providers and individuals alike can work towards better diabetes management and overall well-being.